Lila LEKHAL
Razika BOUKERT

Contribution To The General Study Of The Rat And Its Zoonoses

Lila LEKHAL
Razika BOUKERT

Contribution To The General Study Of The Rat And Its Zoonoses

General Study on the Rat and its Zoonoses

ScienciaScripts

Imprint

Cover image: www.ingimage.com

This book is a translation from the original published under ISBN 978-620-6-72370-7.

Publisher:
Sciencia Scripts
is a trademark of
Dodo Books Indian Ocean Ltd. and OmniScriptum S.R.L publishing group

120 High Road, East Finchley, London, N2 9ED, United Kingdom
Str. Armeneasca 28/1, office 1, Chisinau MD-2012, Republic of Moldova, Europe
Printed at: see last page
ISBN: 978-620-8-14278-0

PEOPLE'S DEMOCRATIC REPUBLIC OF ALGERIA MINISTRY OF HIGHER EDUCATION AND SCIENTIFIC RESEARCH

وزارة التعليم العالي و البحث العلمي

BLIDA1 UNIVERSITY

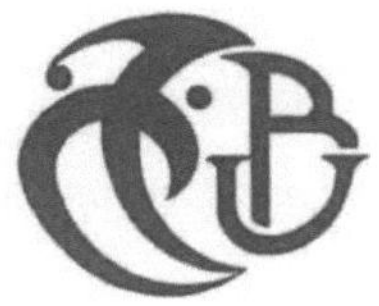

INSTITUTE OF VETERINARY SCIENCES

PRESENTED

DR LEKHAL LILA & DR BOUKERT RAZIKA

CONTRIBUTION TO THE GENERAL STUDY OF THE RAT AND ITS ZOONOSES

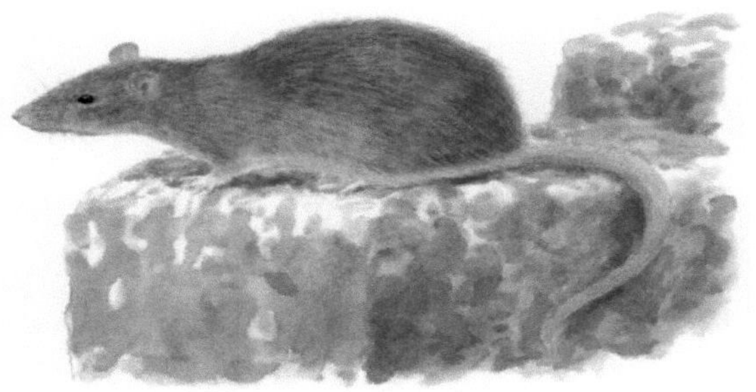

PREAMBLE

This book presents all the knowledge available to date on the rat species and certain related zoonoses. It is intended for veterinary students, veterinary surgeons, technicians and practising veterinarians. It is also intended for public health doctors and technicians, and for municipalities responsible for deratting programmes. It covers the main topics concerning the rat (biology, diversification, deratting, and the main zoonoses, all developed with the help of numerous photos).

Dr LEKHAL L.

Dr BOUKERT R.

TABLE OF CONTENTS

GENERAL INTRODUCTION

Rats are rodents that live in close proximity to humans. These animals compete directly with humans for food, attacking crops and stored products. According to the World Health Organisation (WHO), 20% of the food produced in the world is destroyed by mice/rats. In addition to this damage, the rat can be considered public enemy number 1 for public health, as it is responsible for transmitting more than 40 different types of disease. These include bilharzia, murine typhus, salmonellosis, leptospirosis, trichinellosis, rat-bite fever and bubonic plague, and the mortality associated with the transmission of diseases by rats is very high, It has been estimated that over the last 10 centuries, these diseases have caused more deaths than all the wars that have taken place on the planet, and more recently, up to 10 million deaths have been attributable to rats in the last century alone.

CHAPTER I

GENERAL INFORMATION ON RAT

1.1. Rodents at

Rodents (Rodentia) are an order of mammals, characterised by a dentition consisting of a pair of continuously growing incisors on each jaw. This particular dentition enables them to dig galleries, gnaw their food and defend themselves. 2227 species of rodents exist, occupying the whole planet except Antarctica and a few oceanic islands. The term "rat" is commonly used to designate rodents of the genus Rattus, belonging to the family Muridae, subfamily Murinae, characterised by 3 tuberculated jugal teeth, non-webbed hind limbs and a naked or sparsely hairy tail.

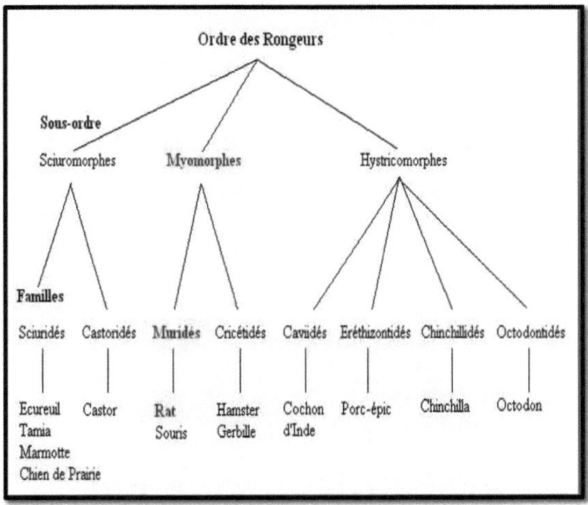

Figure 1: Classification of rodents (Tremblay, 2001).

1.2. The genus Rattus "rat

The genus Rattus (the rat) comprises more than 66 species, most of which are found in South-East Asia and Eurasia, and two which are widespread throughout the world: Rattus Rattus and Rattus Norvegicus. According to Musser and Carlton (2005), species belonging to the genus Rattus can be divided into seven (7) groups:

1. The **Norvegicus** group, comprising Rattus Norvegicus and several other species.

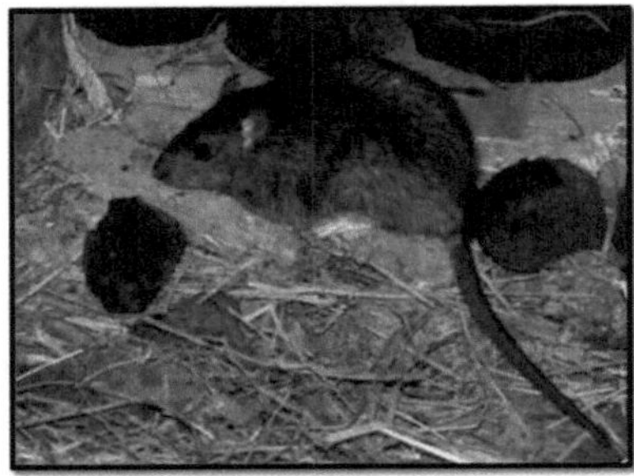

Figure 2: Common names: French: Surmulot - English: Norway Rat - Arabic: Jerd el matha'ib (Ahmim, 2019)

2. The **Exulans** group includes only Rattus Exulans (the Polynesian rat).

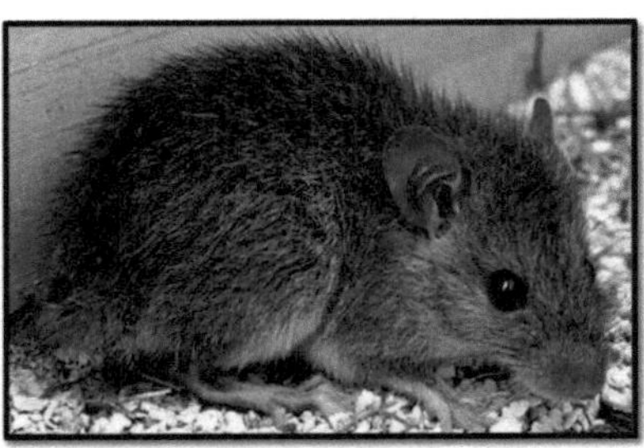

Figure 3: Rattus exulans

(www.cabidigitallibrary.org/doi/10.1079/cabicompendium.46834)

3. The **Rattus** group, comprising Rattus rattus, black rat or roof rat, and Rattus tanezumi (Tanezumi rat), and a large number of related species.

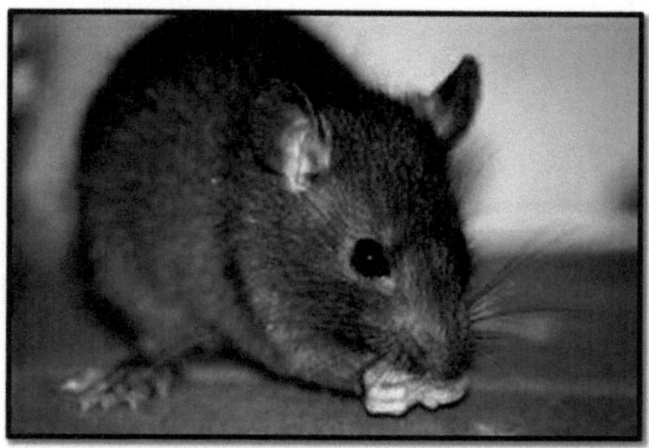

Figure 4: Common names: French: Rat noir - English: Black Rat - Arabic: Jerdoub- Berber: Agherdha (Ahmim, 2019)

4. A **native Australian** group, including Rattus fuscipes (bush rat).

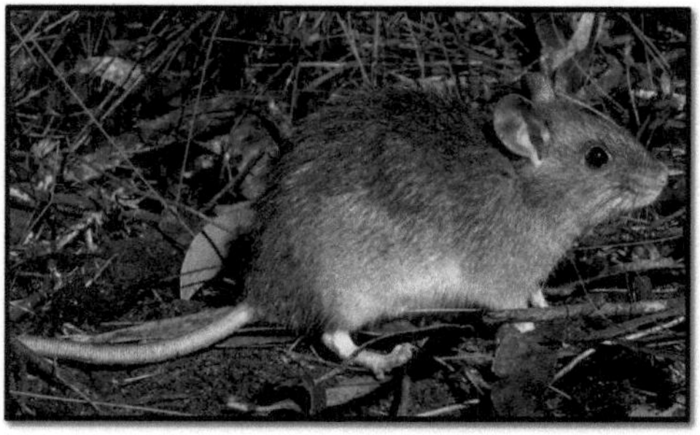

Figure 5: Rattus fuscipes

(https://australian.museum/learn/animals/mammals/bush-rat/)

5. The **New Guinean** group, comprising Rattus leucopus (Cape Cork rat), and Rattus praetor (large New Guinea spiny rat).

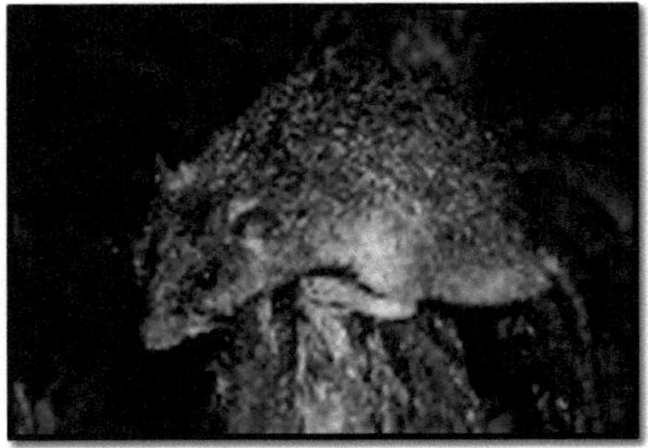

Figure 6: Rattus leucopus https://apps.des.qld.gov.au/species-search/details/?id=742

6. The **Sulawesian** group, comprising Rattus xanthurus (yellow-tailed rat).

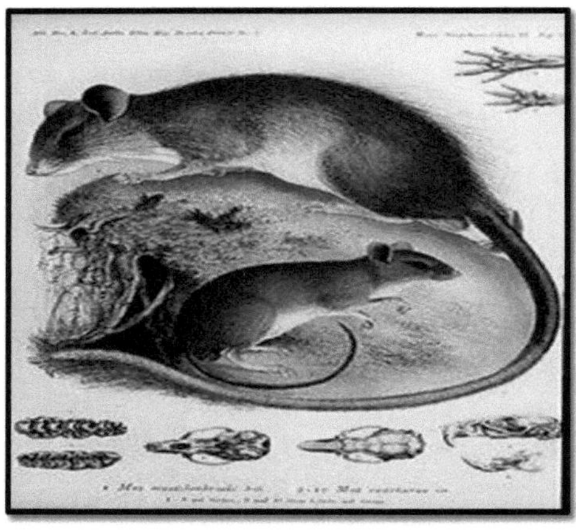

Figure 7: Rattus xanthurus https://animalia.bio/index.php/fr/yellow-tailed-rat

7. The last group includes species belonging to the genus Rattus, whose phylogenetic history has not yet been established.

1.3. General biological data for rats

The main biological data for the rat are given in the table below:

Table 1: Anatomo-physiological data for the rat (Tremblay, 2001).

Longevity	2 to 7 years, 3 years on average
Adult weight female, male	225 to 350g ; 267 to 520g
Birth weight	5 to 6g
Body length	35 to 50 cm
Tail length	17 to 23 cm
Body temperature	35.9 to 38.0°C
Heart rate	250 to 495 beats / min
Respiratory frequency	70 to 145 movements / min
Daily consumption of food for an adult	15 to 20g
Daily water consumption for an adult	22 to 33mL
Daily production of faeces	9 to 15g
Daily diuresis	13 to 23mL

Rats live at an optimum temperature of 22°C, with a temperature range of 18 to 27°C, and a humidity level of 30 to 70%. Rats do not sweat because they have no sweat glands, so they cannot tolerate heat.

1.4. Social structure (Hierarchy)

Rats are social animals, and in their natural habitat, they organise themselves into colonies. Their density remains low, with a single male monopolising the burrow and the females. However, in a richer environment, especially an urban one, the density of rats increases, and they organise themselves into multi-male and multi-female clans, without strict territoriality. However, when young rats reach maturity or when a new congener enters the colony, the dominant individuals benefit more from food and copulation as a result.

1.5. Distribution of activities in space and time

The rat, particularly Rattus Norvegicus, is often regarded as a dirty animal because it lives in sewers and feeds on rubbish. However, this rodent spends 40% of its waking hours in the toilet; it is a clean animal that cleans itself several times a day. Rats are cautious animals, spending around 5% of their time regularly exploring and moving around their environment. Finally, sleep takes up 60% of a rat's time.

1.6. Habitat

The rat is a species of rodent that is genuinely categorised as a human commensal rodent "dependent on man to satisfy its nutritional needs". As a result, it has a significant negative impact on human society and the economy.

1.7. Behaviour

The rat is a myomorphic monogastric rodent that practices coprophagy. It is an omnivore that naturally feeds on leftovers and stocks of food intended for human consumption, and also feeds on small invertebrates, fruit, grains, eggs and grasses. The rat's stomach is small, with a ridge separating the glandular part from the aglandular part, and a resistant cardia. These features of the stomach prevent the rat from vomiting, and force it to divide its meals during the day.

1.8. neophobia

Unlike mice, commensal rats express neophobia. Indeed, on encountering a new food, the rat tends to consume a small quantity, and gradually increase its consumption until it is completely free of this neophobia. Research has shown that rats can even be influenced by the smell of a rat that has ingested a particular food, and also consider an unknown food smelled on the breath of another rat as a known food. Galef et al (1988) showed that this social learning was linked to the presence of carbon disulphide in the breath. In addition, information about food can be transmitted from the mother to her offspring via the mother's milk. Neophobia is also observed in rats during their daily movements i n search of water and food. Rats always follow the same paths, preferring covered routes and lurking in walls.

1.9. Behaviour reproductive

According to Hinds et al (2003), almost millions of rats are born every day in developing countries; indeed, a single pair of rats could be responsible for the birth of more than 3.5 million rats in three years. In both males and females, puberty is reached between 45 and 75 days of age, the The oestrous cycle in females lasts around 4 to 5 days, consisting of 2 days of dioestrus, 12 to 18 hours of prooestrus and then 24 to 36 hours of oestrus. Sexual receptivity lasts around 12 to 20 hours from ovulation, which occurs around 4 to 6 hours after the end of proestrus. In the presence of a single male, the cycles of the females are synchronised (Whitton effect). The rat population is estimated at 1 rat per inhabitant in mainland France, and even 5 rats per inhabitant in Réunion.

1.10. Controlling the rat population

In towns and cities, the annual mortality rate in a rat population is between 91 and 97%. The population reaches equilibrium when the dead are replaced by new births, so the rat population renews itself rapidly.Controlling the rat population in towns used to be based on the use of rat poison following complaints from citizens.Rodenticides are products made from anticoagulants.

The use of anticoagulants was developed in the 1940s. "In addition, rodent populations have developed an acquired genetic resistance to these anticoagulants over time. Recently, a new rodent population control strategy has been adapted (**integrated management programme**), based on a five-stage approach;

1. Identification of the rodent species.

2. Inspection: on-site investigation t o establish control measures.

3. Establishing a tolerance limit; this is the maximum level of infestation tolerated from a health, economic and even aesthetic point of view.

4. Control: reduce the rodent population to an acceptable level by implementing four control measures:

- environmental clean-up measures; public health measures and measures to exclude or prevent access.
- mechanical measures; use of traps to catch rats.
- biological measures, use of predatory species.

- chemical measures; use of rat poison and poisons.

5. Monitoring and evaluation of effectiveness; conducting periodic surveys to estimate the rat population in order to evaluate the management programme adopted and correct it.

Despite the advantages of this management programme, it is cumbersome and costly to implement on the ground, so municipalities and towns tend to control the rat population by using rat poison based on complaints from citizens (a non-integrated programme). Furthermore, incomplete extermination of a rat population can cause a temporary increase in the size of the colony due to massive compensatory reproduction.

CHAPTER II
RATTUS RATTUS ET RATTUS NORVEGICUS

2.1.Origin

The oldest fossils attributed to the genus Rattus have been discovered in Thailand, in Pleistocene sites. The emergence of the genus Rattus dates back to the Middle Pliocene (3.5 million years ago [Ma]), with the species R. norvegicus diverging from an ancestral stock present in Asia 2.8 Ma ago, while the species R. rattus is more recent, dating back 400,000 years. These two invasive species met at a later date, during their respective migrations.

2.1.1. Rattus Rattus

The black rat is thought to have differentiated in India, more specifically the Indian subcontinent, and more particularly the Ganges region and the east coast. The first fossils attributed to R. rattus were discovered in Middle Pleistocene sites in Thailand and Java. The black rat first became a human commensal in the Indus Valley. It was then introduced across the Indian Ocean, the Red Sea and the Mediterranean by Arab ships, reaching Egypt, Turkey and Europe,

In Algeria, historically, in 1858-1867, R. rattus was reported in Bougara (Larbâa), Guellabou (Larbâa), Larbâa (Blida). In 1869, in Guelma. In 1912, in Algiers. In 1937, in Ain Defla, Arrib near Ain Defla, Beni Ounif, Boumedfâa.

2.1.2. Rattus Norvegicus

The brown rat is thought to have originated either in central or southern China, or in northern China and Mongolia, while different, later lineages can be found on every continent.

In Algeria, the surmulot was reported: In 1858, in Algiers, and in 1867 in Mostaganem. In 1885, in EL-Arbâa (Blida). In 1888, in Skikda. In 1932, in Constantine. In 1979, it was reported in the Habibas Islands (Oran), Messerghine, Oran, Ain Temouchent and Es-Sennia.

2.2. Cohabitation between Rattus Rattus and Rattus Norvegicus

the black rat (Rattus rattus) and the brown rat (Rattus norvegicus) seem to have occupied our planet, whether in urban or rural areas.It has also been proven that the invasion of a black rat territory by much larger brown rats forces the latter to leave their nests and take refuge in higher ground, thus no longer benefiting from the food on the ground. The brown rat currently occupies large cities, while the black rat is driven to the outskirts and green spaces.

2.3. Description

2.3.1. Rattus Rattus

Also known as the black rat, this large rodent has a thin, elongated head, well-developed ears and a scaly, hairless tail that is longer than its body. Its thin coat is variable in colour, generally slate-grey on the back, sometimes with a reddish or silvery sheen, and more or less dark grey on the belly, or even yellowish or white. The The skull is globular with curved temporal ridges. It is mainly a nocturnal animal.

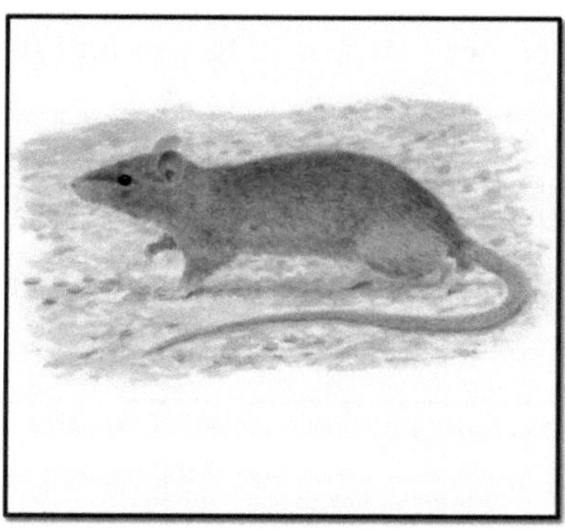

Figure 8: Black Rat (LE BERRE M., 1990)

2.3.2. Rattus Norvegicus

The Norway Warbler is a social species where the family becomes a hierarchical social group. It has a much greater need for humidity than R. rattus and cannot, in particular, do without drinking (even salt water); this limits its range to human habitats in arid areas. It frequents cellars, sewers, canal banks and harbours. It swims well underwater. It is a close commensal of humans. It digs burrows with several entrances, consisting of galleries with reserves and spherical nests. It is active at dusk and dawn.

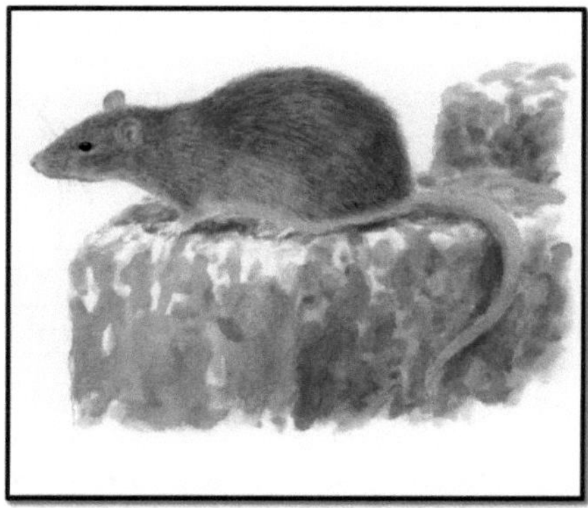

Figure 9: Norway Rat - (LE BERRE M., 1990)

2.4. Morphological difference between R. Rattus and R. Norvegicus

These two species differ morphologically in terms of ear and tail length, body size and slightly different ecological preferences. Recent molecular phylogeny shows that the black rat and the brown rat are not closely related.

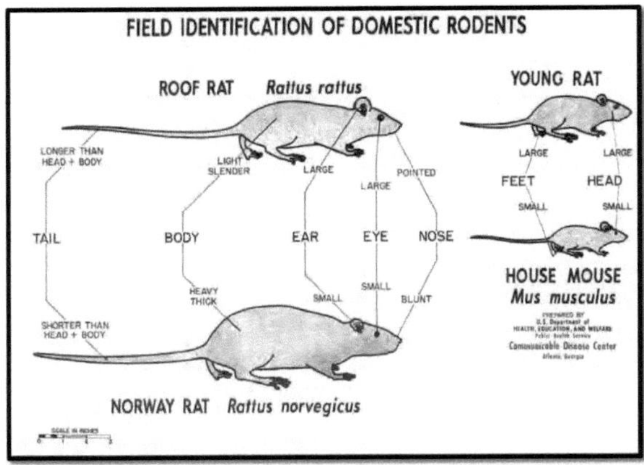

Figure 10: Morphological difference between R. Rattus and R. Norvegicus (http://entomology.ifas.ufl.edu/fasulo/vector/)

R. Rattus and R. Norvegicus can be distinguished in the field by comparing their body measurements: head and body, tail, ear and foot.

Table 2: Body measurements in millimetres for rats **(Ahmmim, 2006)**

	T+C	Q	P	OR
Rattus Rattus	24-27	20,5-21	4-4,3	2-2,3
Rattus Norvegicus	12-20	15-23	2,9-4,2	1,7-2,5

T+C: length of head + body, Q: length of tail, P: length of foot, OR: length of ear.

To measure the head and body, place the animal dorsally, fix the nose with a pin, place a second pin on the side of the anus and measure the distance between the top of the nose and the anus. To measure the length of the tail, measure the distance between the anus and the tip of the tail (figure 11).

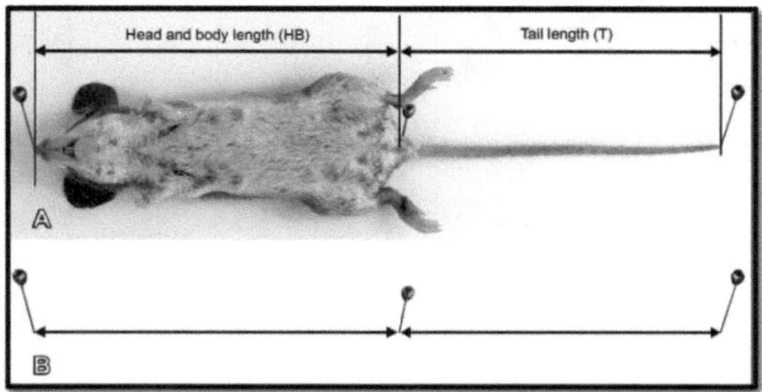

Figure 11: head, body and tail measurements **(Herbreteau, V.; 2011)**

For the foot, measure the distance between the middle toe and the back of the heel (Figure 12).

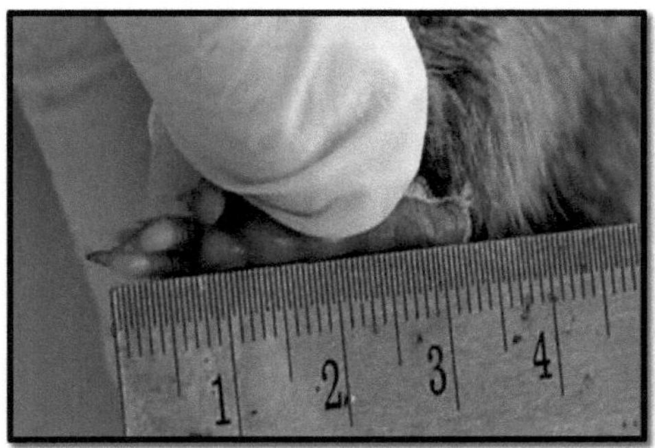

Figure 12: Foot measurements **(Herbreteau, V.; 2011)**

To determine the length of the ear, insert the zero end of the ruler inside the ear and measure the distance between the base and the tip of the ear (Figure 13).

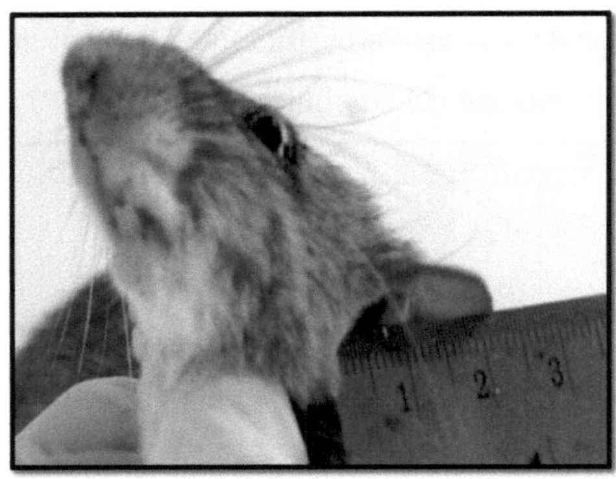

Figure 13: Ear measurement **(Herbreteau, V.; 2011)**

The skull can also be measured using a caliper to compare rodents in general; the distance from the back of the skull to the tip of the nose can be measured (Figure 14).

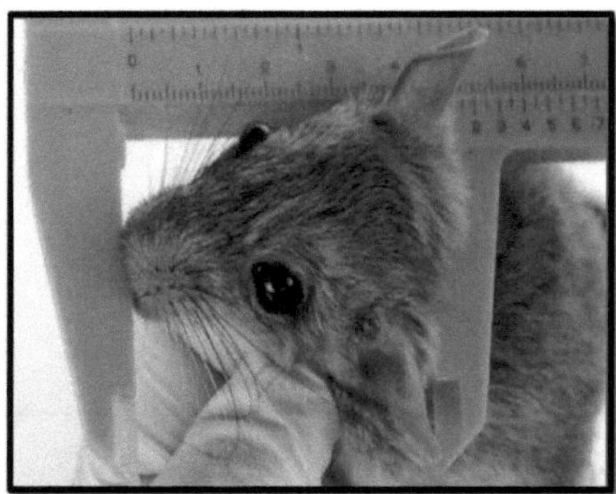

Figure 14: Skull measurements **(Herbreteau, V.; 2011)**

CHAPTER III
RATS AND ZOONOSES

3.1. leptospirosis

Leptospirosis is a re-emerging disease, and is considered to be one of the most widespread infectious diseases in the world. It is also recognised by the WHO as one of the world's neglected tropical diseases, with epidemic potential likely to have a significant impact on public health. Leptospirosis affects more than one million people worldwide, with 60,000 deaths per year. The infection is caused by Leptospira spp. spirochetes, infecting both humans and animals.

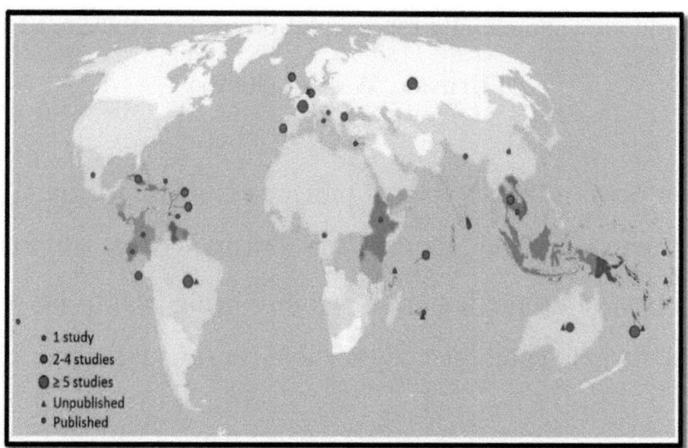

Figure 15: Estimated annual morbidity from leptospirosis worldwide, map published in 2015 - the annual incidence of the disease is represented by an exponential colour gradient from white (0-3), yellow (7-10), orange (20-25) to red (over 100), in cases per 100,000 population. The circles and triangles indicate the country of origin of the published study.

3.1.1. The bacteria

These are the smallest spirochaetes known. Their tips are pointed and one or both are bent into distinctive hook shapes. Depending on the strain, their size varies between 6 and 20 µm long, sometimes more, for a diameter of around 0.1 µm.

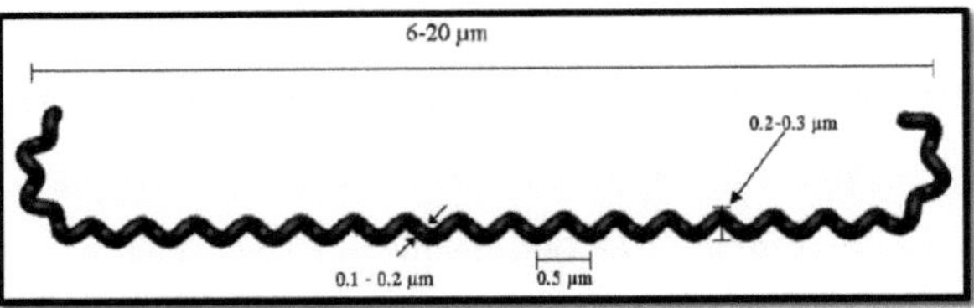

Figure 16: Side view, schematic representation of the structure of Leptospira.

(Jirasak, W et al, 2009)

Leptospires can perform three types of movement: rotation around their central axis, linear progression and circular movements. They are highly mobile bacteria with invasive properties, their mobility being said to be ≪ corkscrew-like ≫ enabling them to enter the body without causing damage or inflammatory reactions.

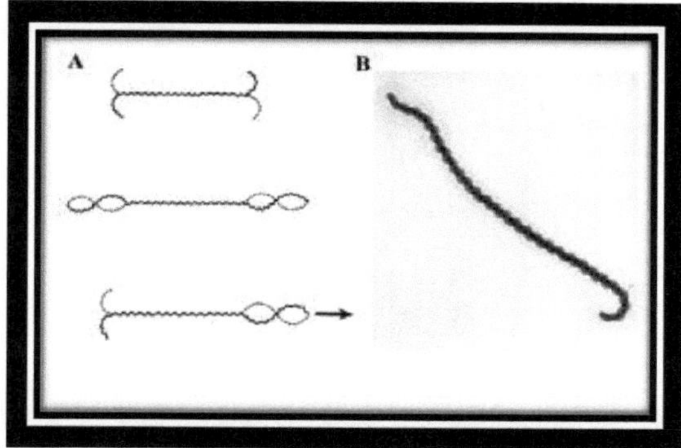

Figure 17: Movement of leptospires (A) **(Charon, N.W et al, 2002)** and electron microscopy of Leptospira biflexa (B) (http://www.pasteur.fr/recherche/Leptospira/Leptospira.html).

3.1.2. Classification of leptospires

3.1.2.1. Classification serological

This classification was established before 1989 and is based on the humoral response induced in an infected individual (production of antibodies).
In this classification, the genus Leptospira is divided into two species:

-Leptospira biflexa (saprophyte)
-Leptospira interrogans (pathogenic)
Species are divided into serovars, which are themselves grouped into serogroups according to their antigenic proximity (Figure 18).

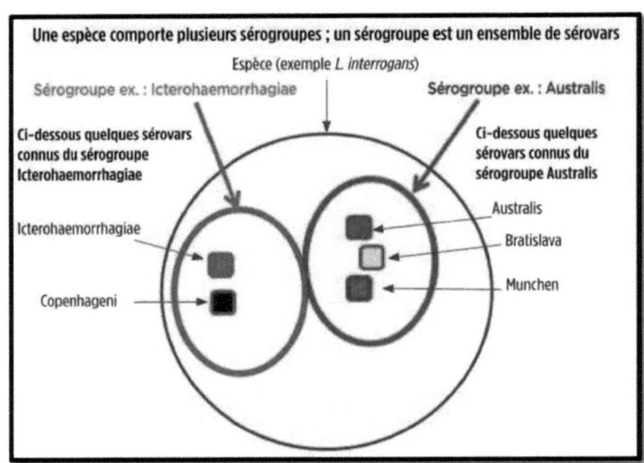

Figure 18: Simplified overview of the systematics of leptospires **(Kodjo, A., 2017)**

Leptospires are divided into more than 250 serovars grouped into more than 32 serogroups.

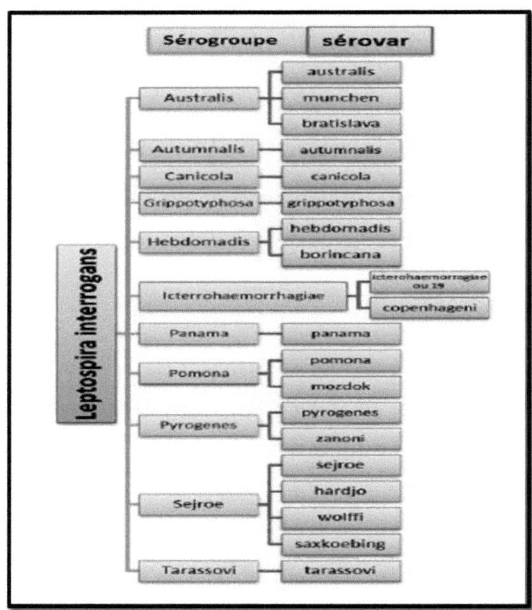

Figure 19: Most important pathogenic serogroups and serovars **(Nennig, M., 2012)**

3.1.2.2. Classification genomics

Since 1987, DNA-DNA hybridisation studies have radically altered the taxonomy of leptospires.Leptospira species are classified on the basis of phylogenetic analyses of DNA sequence data. Leptospira species fall into three groups, comprising pathogens, saprophytes and an intermediate group.

Table 3: Presentation of the genomic species of leptospires described according to their pathogenicity **(Marquez, A., et al, 2017)**

Pathogens	L. interrogans, L. kirschneri, L. borgpetersenii, L. santarosai, L. noguchii, L. weilii, L. alexanderi, L. kmetyi, L. alstonii, L. mayottensis
Intermediaries	L. inadai, L. broomii, L. fainei, L. wolffii, L. licerasiae
Saprophytes	L. biflexa, L. wolbachii, L. meyeri, L. vanthielii, L. terpstrae, L. idonii, L. yanagawae

3.1.3. Reservoirs of leptospires and contamination

The bacterium is maintained in many wild and domestic animal hosts. Rodents, cattle and dogs are considered to be the main source of human infection, but rats are known to be the main source of most cases of human leptospirosis, and are considered to be chronic asymptomatic hosts of Leptospira spp. excreting the bacterium one month after their initial infection with a high concentration of 10^7 leptospires/ml, and reservoirs of L. interrogans in particular. Leptospires infect and persist chronically in the kidneys of reservoir hosts, and are then excreted in the urine, where they can survive for days to months in the environment. Humans are generally contaminated either through contact with carrier animals or contaminated soil, sewage or water.

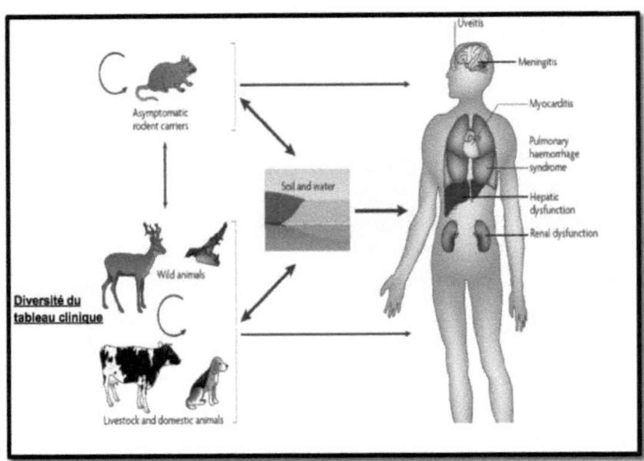

Figure 20: How leptospirosis is transmitted **(Ko, A.I., et al, 2009).**

The survival of leptospires depends on pH, temperature, the possible presence of inhibiting compounds and ultra-violet radiation (direct sunlight). These bacteria can survive for up to three weeks in soggy soil after a rainy season. In soil contaminated with infected rat urine, they can survive for up to two weeks.

Table 4: Survival time of leptospires in different environmental media **(Catalina, P., 2004)**

Tap water, PH 5	2 days
Tap water, pH 7	28 days
Sea water	18-24h
Rubbish	10 days
Wet ground	35 days
Soil saturated with urine	6 months

3.1.4. Human leptospirosis

The average incubation period is one to two weeks (two days to three weeks at the extremes).The clinical expression of leptospirosis is extremely variable. In humans, a benign form is found in 80% of cases, with spontaneous remission, but the infection can lead to severe complications such as renal failure, pulmonary haemorrhage and cardiac complications, with high mortality rates (74%) for pulmonary haemorrhagic syndrome.Generally, leptospirosis is a biphasic disease. The initial acute phase, which lasts about a week, is characterised by the sudden onset of fever, chills, headache, severe myalgias, conjunctival suffusion, anorexia, nausea, vomiting and prostration. However, after a remission of 3 to 4 days the fever may recur, producing a biphasic illness, so Weil syndrome may develop after the acute phase as the second phase of a biphasic illness, or it may simply present as a simple, progressive illness. It is characterised by high fever, intense jaundice, bleeding, renal and pulmonary dysfunction, neurological changes and cardiovascular collapse, with a variable clinical course.

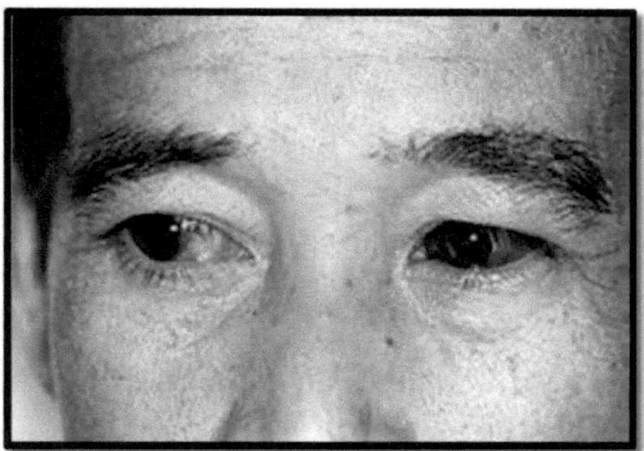

Figure 21: Jaundice-haemorrhagic leptospirosis in humans

In the human population, certain people are particularly at risk of leptospirosis, such as veterinarians, fishermen, butchers and livestock farmers. Vaccinating at-risk populations remains the most viable strategy for controlling this disease, but since vaccine protection is specific to a given serogroup, identifying the strains of leptospires involved in infections is a key factor when setting up a vaccination programme.

3.1.5. Rats and leptospires

Rats are natural reservoirs of leptospires and are considered to be one of the most important sources of leptospirosis, as they are present in abundance in many environments. Pathogenic leptospires were first isolated from wild rats by Noguchi (1917), causing death after inoculation into a guinea pig. Since the first isolation, numerous studies have been carried out to investigate the role of rats in human leptospirosis.Rat infection is well known, and has led to leptospirosis being dubbed the "sewage worker's disease". Indeed, contact with a rat, whatever its zoological species, constitutes an epidemiological risk of the disease.The leptospires penetrate a rat's body, remain in its bloodstream for a variable length of time, and then reach the kidney, which is the target organ. Clinically, the rat presents no symptoms, but the bacteria are regularly eliminated and disseminated in the urine, so a rat can remain infected for many months or even its entire life. Rats are therefore considered to be one of the most important sources of leptospirosis, as they are present in abundance in many environments.The presence of rats around the home has been found to be a risk factor in seropositive patients. Fluctuations in rodent populations can influence the seasonality of leptospirosis. Variations in the incidence of cases may be locally correlated with the rodent breeding season: during the calving season, a large number of young-of-the-year, uninfected rodents may become infected and excrete large quantities of leptospires, leading to a period of high transmission of the bacteria in the rodent population, followed by a peak in the incidence of human cases.How leptospires are transmitted from rat to rat in natural colonies is still unknown. However, urine was the first identified route of excretion of leptospires in rats, discovered at the beginning of the 20th century. It enables leptospires to be transmitted directly through contact with abraded skin or mucous membranes, or through environmental contamination, for example in the case of domestic rat litter or in a town where rats live in close proximity.

Generally Interrogans is the most described genomic species in wild rats (Rattus spp.) worldwide (serovar Icterohaemorrhagiae) and in particular on the African continent (serovar Canicola), other Leptospira species have also been identified in Rattus spp namely, L borgpetersenii, and L. kischneri.

3.2. Bubonic plague

A disease known to be associated with rats, it is caused by Yersinia pestis, a bacterium of the Enterobacteriaceae family. This bacterium was responsible for the deadliest pandemics in human history, the first of which appeared during the sixth and seventh centuries, the second from the fourteenth to the seventeenth centuries, and the third from the nineteenth to the early twentieth centuries. In Algeria, an epidemic of bubonic plague struck the port of Oran in 1556 and 1678, killing 3,000 people. In 1899 the port of Skikda. Three other epidemics were recorded during the nineteenth century: in 1921 (185 cases), in 1931 (76 cases) and in 1944 (95 cases). It used to be thought that it was the brown rat (Rattus Norvegicus) that was responsible for transmitting this disease, but the spread of the disease seems to follow the dispersal of the black rat (Rattus Rattus).

3.2.1. Transmission

In reality, it is not the rat itself that triggers the disease, but rather the fleas (ectoparasites) it carries that are sensitive to the bacteria and responsible for it. For the disease to persist in a region, there must be a wild reservoir (wild rodent) resistant to the bacilli (enzootic), and another living susceptible rodent. Close to humans Following the death of an infected rat, infected fleas leave the corpse of their host in search of another rodent or, failing that, humans. The plague can then be transmitted from human to human.

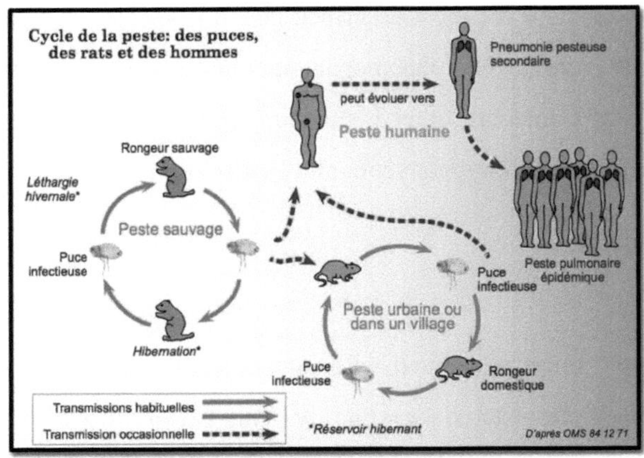

Figure 22: The plague cycle: fleas, rats and humans.

https://books.openedition.org/irdeditions/6604

3.2.2. Symptoms

The incubation period for the disease lasts seven days; after humans are bitten by infected fleas, the bacteria penetrate the body, reaching the lymphatic system and particularly the nearest lymph nodes, where it replicates,At the beginning, a sensation of cold suddenly sets in, followed by hyperthermia which reaches 40°C accompanied by headaches, backache, restlessness, the pulse becomes rapid, these symptoms are followed by prostration, and nervous manifestations such as anxiety, delirium, coma or convulsion, with time, 75-.90% of patients develop a painful swelling of the lymph nodes known as a bubo. At an advanced stage, the inflamed lymph nodes ulcerate and become suppurated, and the disease can spread to the lungs, resulting in the more serious pulmonary form. The fatality rate is between 30 and 60 for the bubonic form, and almost always fatal for the pulmonary form if left untreated.

3.3. Other zoonoses linked to rats

These zoonoses can be transmitted directly from rats to humans, or indirectly via arthropods, farm animals or contaminated food.

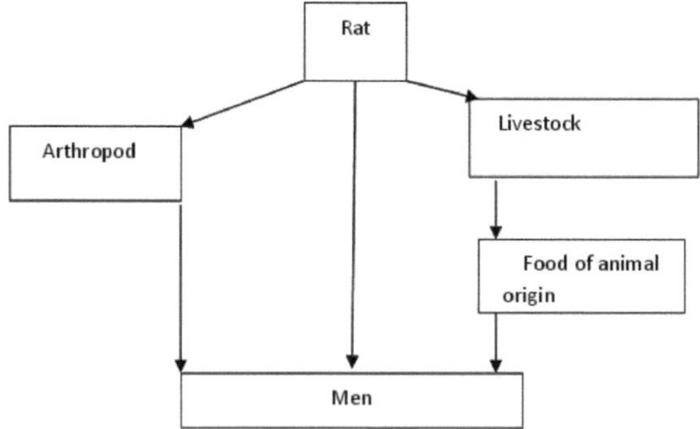

Figure 23: Direct and indirect transmission from rats to humans **(Meerburg B.G et al; 2009)**

Zoonoses linked to rats include :

- Viral zoonoses.
- Bacterial zoonoses.
- Parasitic zoonoses.

These zoonoses are summarised in the tables below according to **(Ayral., F, 2015)**

Table 5: Viral zoonoses

Disease in humans	Agent	Manifestations in rats	Carrier / tank	Manifestations in humans	Mode of transmission in humans
Haemorrhagic fever with renal syndrome	Hantavirus Seoul	NR	tank	Fever, haemorrhage, renal failure	contaminated urine, faeces, saliva
Hepatitis E	Hepatitis E virus	NR	?	acute hepatitis	contaminated food
Poxvirosis	Cowpox virus	NR	tank	skin ulcer	close contact

NR: Not postponed

Table 6: Bacterial zoonoses other than leptospirosis and plague

Disease in humans	Agent	Manifestations in rats	Carrier / tank	Manifestations in humans	Mode of transmission in the man
Murine typhus	Rickettsia typhi	NR	tank	fever, rash, self-limiting	X. cheopsis
Bartonellosis	Bartonella elizabethae + 4 others	NR	tank	fever, endocarditis, neuroretinitis	X. cheopsis
Haverhill fever/ Streptobacillosis or Sodoku	Streptobacillus moniliformis or Spirillum minus	NR	reservoir (commensal bacteria)	fever, rash, polyarthritis, pharyngitis	close contact, bites, contaminated food
Antibiotic-resistant infection	Staph. aureus resistant	NR	portage	skin and soft tissue infection	NR
Antibiotic-resistant infection	Methicillin-resistant Staph. pseudintermedius	NR	portage	skin infection	NR
Tuberculosis	Mycobacterium bovis	Abscess	portage	pneumonia	NR
Colibacillosis	E. coli (O157 STEC)	NR	portage	gastroenteritis	contaminated food
Salmonellosis	Salmonella spp.	NR	tank	gastroenteritis	Soil/water contaminated
Campylobacteriosis	Campylobacter spp.	NR	portage	gastroenteritis	Contaminated soil/water
Yersiniosis	Yersinia Enterocolitica Yersinia pseudotuberculosis	NR	portage	gastroenteritis	Contaminated soil/water
Infection with Clostridium	Clostridium difficile	NR	portage	colitis	Contaminated soil/water

Table 7: Parasitic zoonoses

Disease in humans	Agent	Manifestations in rats	Carrier / tank	Manifestations in humans	Mode of transmission in the man
Cryptosporidiosis	Cryptosporidium spp.	NR	tank	enteritis	contaminated food/water
Toxoplasmosis	Toxoplasma gondii	NR	tank	fever, lymphadenopathy, congenital toxoplasmosis	contaminated food or environment
Trichinellosis	Trichinella spiralis, nematode	NR	tank	gastroenteritis	contaminated pork, raw or undercooked
Angiostrongilosis	Angiostrongilus cantonensis, nematode	granulomatous pneumonia	tank	fever, ocular or meningeal angiostrongilosis	consumption of the paratenic host (mollusc)
Hymenoleiasis	Hymenolepis spp, cestode Rodentolepis spp, cestode	NR	tank	asymptomatic	contaminated food or environment
Hepatic capillariosis	Capillaria hepatica	NR	tank	eosinophilic hepatitis (+/- subclinical)	contaminated food or environment

REFERENCES

1. **Ribeiro do Valle Teixeira, I., Gris, C. F.,** "Genetic diversity of grains, storage pests and their effects on the worldwide bean supply", Nova Science Publishers, In book: Beans: Nutrition, Consumption and Health. 2011 - 353 p.

2. **Battersby, S., Hirschhorn, B.R., Amman, R.B., "Commensal rodents". In Bonnefoy, X., Kampen, H., Sweeney, K.,** "Public health significance of urban pests", Copenhagen, World Health Organization. (2008), 387-419.

3. **Louarn, H. L., Quéré J.P.,** "Les rongeurs de France: faunistique et biologie". Editions Quae. (2003).

4. **Bonnefoy, Xavier, Kampen, Helge, Sweeney,** Kevin & World Health Organization. Regional Office for Europe (2008). Public health significance of urban pests. World Health Organization. Regional Office for Europe. 596p. https://iris.who.int/handle/10665/107363

5. **Saint Girons, M.C.,** "Les Mammifères de France et du Benelux", (Faune Marine Exceptée), Doin, Paris, (1973), 481p.

6. **Tremblay, M.,** "Le Rat", Le jour éditeur, Québec (Collection: Nos amis les animaux), (2001), 175p.

7. **Christiane, C. Denys,** "ORIGIN AND EVOLUTION OF THE BLACK AND BROWN RAT IN EUROPE: A HISTORY OF CO-EVOLUTION? Isabelle
Sidera. Evolutions: Evoluons-nous, Presses Universitaires de Paris Nanterre, 2022, 978-2-84016-512-5.hal 03986828.

8. **Musser, GG., Carlton MD.** 2005. Superfamily Muroidea. In: Wilson DE, Reeder DM (Eds). Mammal Species of the World: A Taxonomic and

Geographic Reference. JHU Press.

9. **Ahmim, M.,** "Les mammifères sauvages d'Algérie Répartition et Biologie de la Conservation". Les Editions du Net, (2019), 978-2312068961. hal-02375326, 289P.

10. **Harkness, J.E. and Wagner, J.E.,** "The biology and medicine of rabbits and rodents", 4th edition Williams & Wilkins compagny, Baltimore, (1995), 372p.

11. **Bauck, L. and Bihun, C.,** "Basic Anatomy, Physiology, Husbandry, and Clinical Techniques" In: Quesenberry K.E., Carpenter J.W. (Eds). "Ferrets, Rabbits, and Rodents: Clinical Medicine and Surgery", Second Edition, Saunders, St Louis, (2004), 286-298.

12. **Berdroy, M. and DrickAmmer, L.,** "Comparative social organization and life history of Rattus and Mus". In: Wolff, J. and Sherman, P., (editors). "Rodent Societies: An Ecological and Evolutionary Perspective", the University of Chicago Press, Chicago, (2007), 610p.

13. **Berdroy, M., Smith, P. and MacDonad, D.,** "Stability of Social Status in Wild Rats: Age and the Role of Settles Dominance", Behaviour, V. 132, n° (3-4), (1995), 193-212.

14. **Wurbel, H., Burn, C. and Latham, N.,** "The Behavior of Laboratory Mice and Rats". In: Jensen, P (editor). "The ethology of domestic animals" 2nd edition: an introductory text. CABI, Cambridge, (2009), 246 p.

15. Bolles, R., "Grooming behavior in the rat", J.Comp. Physiol Psychol, V. 53, n°3, (Jun 1960), 306-310.

16. **Fullerton, H. A. and Berdroy, M.,** "Rats", In: Tynes V (editor). "Behavior of Exotic Pets". Blackwell Publishing, Cambridge, (Augest 2010), 104-116, 248 p.

17. **Modlinska K, Pisula W.,** The Norway rat, from an obnoxious pest to a laboratory pet. Elife. 2020 Jan 17;9:e50651. doi: 10.7554/eLife.50651. PMID: 31948542; PMCID: PMC6968928.

18. **Hurst, J., Bernard, C.J., Hare, R., Whelldon, E.B. and West, C.D.,** "Housing and welfare in laboratory rats: time-budgeting and pathophysiology in single- sex groups". Animal Behaviour, V. 52, n°2, (August 1996), 335-360.

19. **Meyer, A.,** "Urban commensal rodent control: fact or fiction?" In Singleton, R.G., Hinds, A.L., Krebs, J.C., Spratt, M.D. (eds), "Rats, mice and people:rodent biology and management", Canberra, Australian Centre for International Agricultural Research, (2003), 446-450.

20. **Lennox, A. and Bauck, L.,** "Small rodents". In: Quesenberry, K. and Carpenter, J., (editors). "Ferrets, Rabbits and Rodents Clinical Medicine and Surgery", 3rd edition. Elsevier, St Louis, (2011), 608 p.

21. **Galef, B.G. Jr. and Wigmore, S.W.,** (1983) "Transfer of information concerning distant foods": a laboratory investigation of the "information centre" hypothesis. Animal Behaviour, V. 31, n°3, (Augest 1983), 748-758.

22. **Posadas-Andrews, A. and Roper, T.J.,** "Social transmission of food preferences in adult rats", Animal Behaviour, V. 31, n°3, (February 1983), 265-271.

23. **Galef, B., Mason, J., Preti, G. and Bean, N.,** "Carbon Disulfide: A Semiochemical Mediating Socially-Induced Diet Choice in Rats". Physiol Behav, V. 42, n°2, (1988), 119-124.

24. **Galef, B.G. Jr. and Clark, M.M.**, "Mother's milk and adult presence: two factors determining initial dietary selection by weanling rats", Journal of Comparative and Physiological Psychology, V. 78, n°2, (February 1972), 220-225.

25. **Bond, N.W.,** "The poisoned partner effect in rats: some parametric considerations". Animal Learning and Behaviour, V. 12, n°1, (March1984), 89-96.

26. **Hepper, P.G.,** "Fetal olfaction". In: MacDonald DW, Muller-Schwarze D, Natynczuk SE, eds. "Chemical signals in vertebrates. Oxford, Oxford University Press: (1990), 282-287.

27. **Lanoix J. N. and Roy M. L.,** "Manuel du technicien sanitaire", World Health Organization, Geneva, (1976), 193p.

28. **Fortin A.,** "VERS UNE GESTION PLUS EFFICACE ET DURABLE DES RATS EN MILIEU URBAIN", MAITRISE EN ENVIRONNEMENT UNIVERSITÉ DE SHERBROOKE, 2012.

29. **Hinds, L.A., Hardy, C.M., Lawson, M.A. and Singleton, G.R.,** "Developments in Fertility Control For Pest Animal Management. In: Rats, Mice and People: Rodent Biology and Management, Singleton, G.R., Hinds, C.J. Krebs and Spratt, D.M., (Eds), ACIAR Monograph, Australia (2003), 31-36.

30. **Bridier, E., Aure, F., Mottier, F., Nivet, A., Lai-Man, G. and Boyer, N.,** "Les rongeurs à la Réunion, sources de nombreux fléaux", Phytoma Déf. Vég, V. 595, (July 2006), 9-12.

31. **Davis, D.E.,** "The Characteristics of Rat Populations", Quart. Rev. Biol, V. 28, n°4, (December 1953), 373-401.

32. **Twigg, G.,** The brown rat. Devon, David & Charles (Holdings) Ltd, (1975), 150p.

33. **Sarisky, P.J., Hirschhorn, B.R. and Baumann, J.G.** (2008). Integrated pest management. In Bonnefoy, X., Kampen, H. and Sweeney, K., Public health significance of urban pests (pp. 543-562). Copenhagen, World Health

Organization. ISBN # 978-92-890-7188-8

34. **Flint, M. and Gouveia, P.** (2001). The integrated pest management concept. In ARN Publications, IPM in pratice - Principles and methods of integrated pest management (p. 31-52). Okland, California, Library of congress.

35. **Greaves, J.H., Hammond, L.E. and Bathard, A.H.,** "The control of re-invasion by rats of part of a sewer network", The Annals of Applied Biology, V. 62, n°2, (October 1968), 341-351.

36. **Barnett, S.A.,** "The rat: a study in behavior"**.** Chicago, University of Chicago Press, (1975).

37. **Ahmim, M.,** "Les mammifères d'Algérie des origines à nos jours", (2004), pages 199, 200, 203 and 206.

38. **LE BERRE M.,** 1990 - Fauna of the Sahara - Mammals. Raymond CHABAUD - LECHEVALIER, T. 2, 360 p.

39. Public Health Pesticide ApplicatorTraining Manual index, http://entomology.ifas.ufl.edu/fasulo/vector/.

40. **Herbreteau, V.; Jittapalapong, S.; Rerkamnuaychoke, W.; Chaval, Y.; Cosson, J.F.; Morand, S.** "Protocols for Field and Laboratory Rodent Studies"; Kasetsart University: Bangkok, Thailand, 2011; p. 51.

41. **Hartskeerl, R. A., Collares-Pereira, M., & Ellis, W. A.,** "Emergence, control and reemerging leptospirosis: dynamics of infection in the changing world", Clinical Microbiology and Infection, V.17 n°4, (2011), 494-501.

42. **Levett, P.N.,** "Leptospirosis", Clinical Microbiology Reviews, V. 14, n°2, (April 2001), 296-326.

43. World Health Organization. The control of neglected zoonotic diseases: from advocacy to action: report of the fourth international meeting held at WHO

Headquarters, Geneva, Switzerland, 19-20 November 2014. (2015). http://apps.who.int/iris/handle/10665/183458

44. **Costa, F., Hagan, J.E., Calcagno, J., Kane, M., Torgerson, P., Martinez-Silveira, M.S., et al.** "Global Morbidity and Mortality of Leptospirosis: A Systematic Review", PLoS Negl Trop Dis V. 9, (2015), e0003898.

45. **Vinetz J.M, Watt.G.,** "79 - Leptospirosis", Hunter's Tropical Medicine and Emerging Infectious Diseases (Tenth Edition), 2020, 636-640.

46. **Bomfim, M.R.Q., Barbosa-Stancioli, E.F., Koury. M.C.,** "Detection of pathogenic leptospires in urine from naturally infected cattle by nested PCR", Vet J, V. 178 (2007), 251-6.

47. **Jirasak Wong-ekkabut, Sudarat Chadsuthi, Wannapong Triampo, Galayanee Doungchawee, Darapond Triampo and Chartchai Krittanai,** "Leptospirosis research: Response of pathogenic spirochete to ultaviolet-A irradiation", African Journal of Biotechnology, V. 8, no. 14, (20 July, 2009), 3341-3352.

48. Bharti, A.R., Nally, J.E., Ricaldi, J.N., Matthias, M.A., Diaz, M.M., Lovett,M.A., Levett, P.N., Gilman, R.H., Willig, M.R., Gotuzzo, E. and Vinetz, J.M. on behalf of the Peru-United States Leptospirosis Consortium, "Leptospirosis: a zoonotic disease of global importance", the Lancet infectious disease,V. 3, n° 12, (December 2003), 757-771.

49. **Legrand, E.,** "La leptospirose bovine", Thèse d'exercice vétérinaire, Doctorat Vétérinaire Faculté De Médecine De Creteil, Alfort, (2007).

50. **Charon, N.W. and Goldstein S.F.,** "Genetics of motility and chemotaxis of a fascinating group of bacteria: The Spirochetes", Annu Rev Genet, V. 36, (Jun 2002), 47-73.

51. INSTITUT PASTEURFrance
:http://www.pasteur.fr/recherche/Leptospira/Leptospira.html.

52. **Adler, B. and de la Peña Moctezuma, A.,** "Leptospira and leptospirosis", Veterinary Microbiology, V. 140, n° 3-4, (January 2010), 287-296.

53. **Kodjo, A.,** "Prerequisites for the biological diagnosis of canine leptospirosis," PratiqueVet, vol. 52, (2017), pp. 146-149.

54. **Caimi, K., & Ruybal, P.** (2020). "Leptospira Spp. a genus in the stage of diversity and genomic data expansion. Infection, Genetics and Evolution": Journal of Molecular Epidemiology and Evolutionary Genetics in Infectious Diseases, 81, 104241. 10.1016/j.meegid.2020.104241

55. **Nennig, M.,** Profil sérologique et recherche de leptospires pathogènes par méthode PCR sur sang et urine de chiens apparemment sains : étude prospective sur 30 cas. (2012), http://portaildoc-veto.vetagrosup. en/?q=node/122.

56. **Brenner, D.J., Kaufmann, A.F., Sulzer, K.R., Steigerwalt, A.G., Rogers, F.C. and Weyant, R.,** "Further determination of DNA relatedness between serogroups and serovars in the family Leptospiraceae with a proposal for Leptospira alexanderi sp. nov. and four new Leptospira genomospecies", International Journal of Systematic Bacteriology, V. 49, n° Pt 2, (April 1999), 839-858.

57. **Xu, Y., Zhu, Y., Wang, Y., Chang, Y.F., Zhang, Y., Jiang, X., Wang, J.,** (2016). "Whole genome sequencing revealed host adaptation-focused genomic plasticity of pathogenic Leptospira", Scientific Reports, 6. (2016).

58. **Marquez, A., Djelouadji, Z., Lattard, V., and A. Kodjo, A.,** "Overview of laboratory methods to diagnose Leptospirosis and to identify and to type leptospires", Int. Microbiol, vol. 20, no. 4, (2017), pp. 184-193.

59. **Boey, K., Shiokawa, K., Rajeev, S.,** "Leptospira infection in rats: A literature review of global prevalence and distribution, PLoS Negl Trop Dis, V. 13, (2019), e0007499.

60. **Ko, A.I., Goarant, C., Picardeau, M.,** "Leptospira: the dawn of the molecular genetics era for an emerging zoonotic pathogen", Nat Rev Microbiol, V. 7, n°10, (2009), 736-47.

61. **Ayral, F., Artois, J., Zilber, A.L., Widen, F., Pounder, K.C., Aubert, D., and Atrois, M.,** "The relationship between socioeconomic indices and potentially zoonotic pathogens carried by wild Norway rats: Asurvey in Rhône, France (2010-2012)", Epidemiology and Infection, V. 143 n°3, (2015), 586-599.

62. **Trueba, G., Zapata, S., Madrid, K., Cullen, p., Haake, D.,** "Cell aggregation a mechanism of pathogenic Leptospira to survive in fresh water", Inte Microbiol,
V. 7, (2004), 35-40.

63. **Chang, S.L., Buckingham, M., Taylor, M.P.,** "Studies on Leptospira icterohaemorrhagiae; survival in water and sewage; destruction in water by halogen compounds, synthetic detergents, and heat", J Infect Dis, V. 82 n°3, (May-June 1948), 256-66.

64. **Catalina, P.,** "Leptospirosis and companies. Conduite à tenir" (2004), 5p.

65. Guerra, M.A., "Leptospirosis", Journal of American Veterinary Medical Association, V. 234, n° 4, (February 2009), 472-478.

66. **Perolat, P.,** LEPTOSPIRA - Medical Bacteriology Course. 2003. Université Médicale Virtuelle Francophone (UMVF) - Université Paris Descartes (12/02/2020). http://www.microbes-edu.org/etudiant/Leptospira.

67. **Dolhnikoff, M., Mauad, T., Bethlem, E. P., Carvalho, C. R.,** "Pathology and pathophysiology of pulmonary manifestations in leptospirosis", Brazilain Journal of Infectious Diseases, V. 11, (2007), **142-148**.

68. World Health Organization (WHO). 2003. Human Leptospirosis: Guidance for Diagnosis, Surveillance and Control. Geneva, Switzerland:

http://www.who.int/csr/don/en/WHO_CDS_CSR_EPH_2002.23.pdf.

69. **Yinghua, Xu, Qiang, Ye,** "Human leptospirosis vaccines in China", Hum Vaccin Immunother, V. 14 n°4, (2018), 984-993.

70. Leptospirosis, "information and treatments", Institut Pasteur France, (2018).

71. **Mohamed-Hassan, S.N., Bahaman, A.R. Mutalib and Khairani-Bejo, S.,** "Prevalence of Pathogenic Leptospires in Rats from Selected Locations in Peninsular Malysia", Research Journal of Animal Sciences, V. 6, n°1, (2012), 12-25.

72. **Vintz, J.M., G.E. Glass, C.E. Flexner, P. Mueller and D.C. Kaslow,** "Sporadic urban leptospirosis", Ann.Intern.Med, V. 125, n° 10, (November 1996), 794-798.

73. **KOSSEY-VRAIN, C.,** "La leptospirose canine: revue bibliographique", Med. Vét. ENVA, N°135, (2004), 150p.

74. **Barcellos, C., Lammerhirt, C.B., de Almeida, M.A.B. and dos Santos, E.,** "Spatial distribution of leptospirosis in Rio Grande do Sul, Brazil: recovering the ecology of ecological studies", Cad Saude Publica, V. 19, n° 5, (Sept-Oct 2003), 1283-1292.

75. **Davis, S., Calvet, E. and Leirs, H.,** "Fluctuating rodent populations and risk to humans from rodent-borne zoonoses", Vect Borne Zoo Dis, V. 5, n°4, (Winter 2005), 305-314.

76. **Holt, J., Davis, S. and Leirs, H.,** "A model of leptospirosis infection in an African rodent to determine risk to humans: seasonal fluctuations and the impact of rodent control", Acta Trop, V. 99, n° (2-3), (October 2006), 218-225.

77. **Villanueva, S. Y. A. M., M. Saito, R. A. Baterna, C. A. M. Estrada, A. K. B. Rivera, M.C. Dato et al.** "Leptospira-Rat-Human Relationship in Luzon, Philippines". Microbes and Infection / Institut Pasteur, V. 16, n° 11, (2014), 902-10.

78. **Ido, Y., Hoki, R., Ito, H. and Wani H.,** "The rat as a carrier of Spirochaeta icterohaemorrhagiae, the causative agent of Weil's disease (Spirochaetosis icteohaemorrhagica)", J Exp Med, V 26, n° 3, (September 1917), 341-353.

79. Gaudie, C. M., Featherstone, C. A., Phillips, W. S., McNaught ,R., Rhodes,P. M., Errington, J., et al. "Human Leptospira Interrogans Serogroup Icterohaemorrhagiae Infection (Weil's Disease) Acquired from Pet Rats". The Veterinary Record, V. 163, No. 20, (2008), 599-601.

80. **Inge, M. Krijger, Ahmed A. A. Ahmed, Marga G. A. Goris, Peter W. G. Groot Koerkamp, and Bastiaan G. Meerburg,;** "Prevalence of Leptospira Infection in Rodents from Bangladesh" nt. J. Environ. Res. Public Health. 2019, 16-2113.

81. **Houemenou, G., Ahmed, A., Libois, R., Hartskeerl, R. A.,** "Leptospira spp. Prevalence in Small Mammal Populations in Cotonou, Benin". Hindawi Publishing Corporation ISRN Epidemiology, V. 2013, (2013), Article ID 502638, 8 pages.

82. **Perry, RD, and Fetherston, JD,** "Yersinia pestis-etiologic agent of plague", Clin Microbiol Rev, 10(1), 35, 1997.

83. **Bastiaan G Meerburg, Grant R Singleton, and Aize Kijlstra,** "Rodent-borne diseases and their risks for public health", Critical Reviews in Microbiology, 2009; 35(3): 221-270.

84. Health bulletin. Gouvernorat General de l'Algérie. 1909-1941. p. 94-524.

85. **Mafart B, Brisou P, Bertherat E.** Epidemiology and management of plague epidemics in the Mediterranean during the Second World War. Bull Soc Pathol Exot. 2004;97:306-10.

86. World health Organisation www.who.int/fr/news-room/fact-sheets/detail/plague.

87. **Ayral, F.,** "Vers une surveillance des zoonoses associées aux rats (Rattus Norvegicus), PhD thesis from Grinoble Alpes University, May 2015.

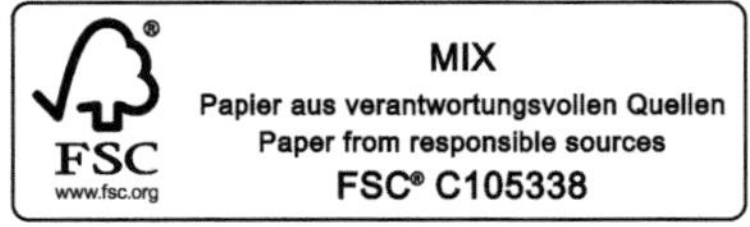

Printed by Books on Demand GmbH, Norderstedt / Germany